A

Blueprint For Women, Diet and Hormones

A

Comprehensive Four-Week

On How To Achieve Hormonal Balance

And Lose Weight

Elizabeth Kettner, MD

Disclaimer

This publication is designed to provide accurate, reliable, and authoritative information regarding the subject matter covered. The author and publisher do not assume any responsibility for errors, inaccuracies, or omissions.

By its sale, neither the publisher nor the author is engaged in rendering or other professional services. If expert assistance and guidance are needed, the services of a competent and skillful professional should be sought.

CONTENTS

AUTHOR'S NOTE

Women come to me feeling overtired, grumpy, stressed and inevitably regretting the extra pounds they've put on despite their best attempts to exercise and eat correctly. This is something that I've seen time and time again in my practice, and it's something that I've seen quite a few times. When women reach the middle of their thirties, they are more likely to begin experiencing these conditions. It is becoming increasingly difficult for my patients to keep their weight at a healthy level. Even with the discipline that January provides, it is more difficult to lose those pounds that you gained on Holi. It would appear that the diet regimens that were successful in the past are no longer effective. What is even more depressing is the fact that diets that are successful for male coworkers and spouses do not appear to be successful for them.

When I explain to my patients that the solution to their problems is not to be found by counting calories or clocking kilometers on the treadmill, but rather by learning to understand the language of hormones, they are frequently astonished by my explanation.
What are you thinking? Are you referring to hormones? Yes, hormones. I can assist you in doing exactly that by utilizing science that respects your body.

What does that mean, exactly? When your diet and lifestyle support your hormones, your hormones will support you. When your body receives instructions from the food you eat to burn fat and promote health, it is like a refreshing breeze on a hot summer day. You turn a metabolic switch, and your body is altered. This is particularly welcome after age thirty-five when the scale is tougher to budge!

What makes the scale stick? Your metabolism is grinding to a standstill. Your metabolism is the sum of all of the biochemical reactions in your body, including those connected to your hormones, that control how you feel and decide how fast or slow you burn calories. Metabolism is the cornerstone of your health, today and tomorrow. When you learn to speak the language of hormones, you may enhance your metabolism, shed fat, and finally maintain a healthy body weight by burning rather than storing fat. At the same time, you eliminate nagging, unpleasant symptoms including weariness, cravings, moodiness, insomnia, and a poor immune system. Too many health programs don't function because they are developed by men, for men, and not for women's complicated hormonal demands. I'm going to show you how to reach this ultimate aim in a way that honors your unique female DNA.

WHAT YOU SHOULD EAT?

Many of my patients want to know what to eat to keep healthy, yet they feel confused. And over time, the answer has evolved. As fasting protocols became all the rage, the focus changed from what should I eat to when should I eat. Very frequently my sufferers come to me having attempted those numerous plans, simplest to locate they simply won weight, or they're so beaten with choices, they live in the same food rut because they aren't sure which plan is suitable for them.

What not to eat is easy. The reality is, that a powerful correlation exists between intake of processed food, weight increase, and low immunity. More than half of Americans' calorie consumption now comes from ultra-processed foods: chips, soda, cookies, candy, and other Franken foods. The consequences are obvious to see. Not only did the United States do worse than many other countries during the COVID-19 epidemic, but also our rates of weight gain, obesity, diabetes, cardiovascular disease, cancer, and depression are high. The stuff we eat sets us up to be traordinarily sick, rendering us subject to chronic disease and viruses like COVID-19.

Eat for your hormones.

Food is the backbone of the hormones you create. When it comes to your health and metabolism, food is medication. I'm going to clear up the confusion about what's healthy and what's not and offer you all the assistance you need to be successful. I'll provide a proven regimen that's designed to fit your hormonal demands and help you restore your health in four weeks. To start, ingesting healthy fat is very crucial to long-term hormone balance. Healthy fat makes you feel more satisfied, and it slows down or eliminates the surges in blood sugar that might cause you to accumulate fat. You need reasonable protein not so much that it turns into sugar, but not so little that your muscles start to break down. Some principles you've certainly heard about previously are vital too, such as avoiding sugar and excess processed carbohydrates, enjoying healthy fats like extra-virgin olive oil and avocado oil, and even following fasting protocols. I've incorporated these tactics into a single cohesive strategy I call the Gottfried Protocol, which will allow you to flip your metabolism from stuck and inflexible to unstuck and flexible. As you do so, you'll lengthen your health span (that is, your healthy life span), support your immune system, and improve your general health.

WHAT YOU SHOULD KNOW ABOUT NUTRITION?

I didn't learn the answers to these dietary inquiries at Harvard Medical School or the University of California at San Francisco, where I served my internship and residency in obstetrics and gynecology. In reality, during my medical school, nutrition and lifestyle approaches to health were tolerated but never championed.

Yet this lack of attention constituted a scientific contradiction that has since been evolving. We now know that better nutrition and lifestyle are the most essential drivers of illness pre-prevention and reversal for the people who are prepared to commit to them. Science has documented the evidence for this reality many times over, yet the discoveries have been generally ignored by orthodox medicine.

Look no further than the hormone insulin. You've probably heard of it. Insulin's principal duty is to transfer glucose into your cells, thereby reducing the glucose in your blood. It's an important hormone in the treatment and prevention of diabetes. The scientific literature demonstrates that dietary and lifestyle approaches to diabetes a condition in which cells become numb to the hormone insulin work better than medications, perhaps because they don't disrupt normal chemistry and instead help an individual return to a state of homeostasis, or balance. Yet few clinicians (myself included) taught how to employ dietary intervention or how to support changes to behavior and lifestyle.
As a result, I had to teach myself how to accomplish these things. Fortunately, I had an excellent patient, one who struggled with various hormone problems: me. My effort to balance my hormones has informed my profession as a physician and writer.
In medical school, I was trained to counsel patients to exercise more and eat less if they wished to reduce weight. When I followed that advice, I made my hormone imbalance worse be- cause the critical role of metabolic hormones, and how they act in women, was absent from the equation.

In my twenties, I began to fight melancholy, premenstrual symptoms, and belly obesity. I fought with my weight because my levels of testosterone, growth hormone, estrogen, and progesterone were too low, and my insulin and cortisol were too high. That made me get stressed over the small stuff. I'd work out for hours with nothing to show for it on the bathroom scale or in my muscles. I was on a primarily vegan diet, and I wasn't getting the healthful fat I required to manufacture these hormones in my body. Seemingly overnight, my triceps area turned flabby. There were longitudinal lines on my nails, and I spotted bizarre fatty "cushions" at my knees. What?! Worst of all, I felt stressed and overwhelmed much of the time; I lacked inner calm. Instead, you may observe difficulty with sleeping, with reducing the baby's weight, or with reduced sex drive. Maybe your workouts don't seem to have an impact.
After being prescribed an antidepressant and the birth control pill to address my problems, I just felt they were not the correct treatment. Then, with a simple blood test, I learned my hormones were out of balance. As I addressed my hormones, I found they were the fundamental source of my difficulties. I began finding hormone imbalances in practically all of my patients who were drugged by their well-meaning doctors. I wrote numerous books about how to balance hormones: The Hormone Cure, The Hormone Reset Diet, Younger, and Brain Body Diet. My purpose is to save you time in finding a solution. I identified what worked, and what didn't, to get my hormones back in the target zone, burn fat, and lose weight. You can too.

Thankfully, the culture of medicine is evolving. Science and technology are advancing. My practice has transformed, thanks to these recent advancements.

Today I help my patients personalize the way they eat into their hormones. Defined by the National Institutes of Health as a developing approach to illness treatment and prevention, precision medicine takes into account individual heterogeneity in genes, environment, and lifestyle. This is a collaborative approach involving the patient and other professionals; we share a single dashboard monitoring health and development.

Do you need to go that far to reduce weight and get healthier? Not necessarily. But the material and experience that I built up over the past five years while coaching patients through my procedures are now simplified into the book you're holding and the four-week program you will learn.

PART I: Navigating the Intricate Symphony: An In-Depth Introduction to Hormones

We would like to take this opportunity to welcome you to the beginning of our adventure, which is into the complex world of hormones, which are the messengers that conduct the symphony of our body's operations. In the course of this in-depth investigation, we will delve deeply into the scientific principles that underlie hormones, gaining knowledge of the crucial function that hormones play in preserving equilibrium, influencing our health, and sculpting our general well-being. In preparation for the unraveling of the intriguing tapestry of hormones, which are the unseen conductors that are orchestrating the intricate dance that occurs within.

Exposing the Hormonal Ensemble to the Public
An Explanation of This Concept Hormones
The glands that are part of the endocrine system are responsible for the production of hormones, which are signaling molecules that are then delivered directly into the bloodstream to regulate physiological processes. Consider them to be messengers who travel through the extensive communication network of your body, passing on vital instructions to the organs and tissues that are responsible for their function.

The Endocrine System:
A Command and Control Center with
The pituitary gland, thyroid gland, adrenal glands, and reproductive glands are all examples of glands that are part of the endocrine system. Imagine the endocrine system as a sophisticated command center. These glands work in unison, secreting hormones that pass via the circulation to target cells, guaranteeing optimal functioning and equilibrium.

The Dance of Key Hormones
Insulin: The Blood Sugar Maestro
Produced by the pancreas, insulin serves a crucial function in regulating blood sugar levels. It lets cells absorb glucose for energy, maintaining a delicate balance necessary for overall health. Dysregulation of insulin can lead to illnesses like diabetes.

Thyroid Hormones: Metabolic Maestros
Thyroid hormones, particularly thyroxine (T4) and triiodothyronine (T3) are crucial participants in metabolism. They influence energy production, body temperature, and even weight regulation. Imbalances can lead to illnesses such as hypothyroidism or hyperthyroidism.

Estrogen and Progesterone: Orchestrating Reproduction
These hormones, largely produced by the ovaries, influence the menstrual cycle, pregnancy, and overall reproductive health in women. Beyond reproduction, they affect mood, bone health, and cardiovascular function.

Testosterone: More Than a Male Hormone
While testosterone is frequently associated with masculine development, it's found in both men and women. It affects muscular mass, bone density, libido, and even mood. Maintaining a balance is vital for general well-being.

Cortisol: The Stress Conductor
Produced by the adrenal glands, cortisol is the body's major stress hormone. It helps regulate metabolism and plays a part in the body's fight-or-flight response. Chronic stress can lead to cortisol abnormalities, impacting different physical functions.

The Symphony of Hormonal Communication
Hormone Receptors: Receiving the Melody
Each hormone has particular receptors on target cells, comparable to locks and keys. When a hormone attaches to its receptor, it begins a cascade of actions, delivering the hormonal message and evoking the proper reaction from the cell.

Negative Feedback Loops: Maintaining Harmony
To prevent hormonal pandemonium, the body develops negative feedback loops. When hormone levels reach a specific threshold, the body signals the glands to halt or terminate hormone production, ensuring a delicate balance is maintained.

Influencing Factors: Nature and Nurture
Genetic Factors
Genetics plays a key part in shaping an individual's hormonal constitution. Genetic differences can alter hormone synthesis, receptor sensitivity, and total hormonal responsiveness.

Lifestyle and Environmental Factors
External factors, such as nutrition, stress levels, sleep patterns, and exposure to environmental contaminants, can drastically alter hormone equilibrium. Understanding these impacts helps individuals to make informed lifestyle choices.

Hormones Across the Lifespan
Hormones in Development
From embryonic development until puberty, hormones guide the delicate process of growth, maturation, and sexual development. The choreographed ballet of hormones molds our bodies and prepares us for maturity.

Hormones in Adulthood
As we grow into adulthood, hormones continue to play critical functions in sustaining reproductive health, metabolism, and overall well-being. Understanding these relationships is crucial to proactive health management.

Hormones in Aging
The aging process brings about hormonal changes, including menopause in women and andropause in men. Navigating these transitions demands a detailed grasp of hormonal fluctuations and their health implications.

Hormonal Imbalances and Health Implications
Common Hormonal Disorders
Disruptions in hormonal balance can lead to different illnesses, such as diabetes, hypothyroidism, polycystic ovarian syndrome (PCOS), and adrenal insufficiency. Recognizing symptoms and seeking appropriate action is crucial for effective management.

Impact on Mental Health
Hormones regulate neurotransmitters and brain function, having a role in mental health problems such as sadness and anxiety. A holistic approach to mental well-being includes treating hormonal variables.

Hormones and Gender Identity
Beyond Binary Perspectives
Understanding hormones extends to understanding and appreciating varied gender identities. Hormonal therapies play a significant part in gender-affirming care, matching an individual's physical body with their gender identification.

For transgender individuals, hormone treatments are not just physical but also psychological. Navigating the mental health components of gender-affirming care demands a sensitive and holistic approach.

Practical Implications and Takeaways
Holistic Health Practices
Maintaining hormonal balance needs holistic strategies spanning nutrition, stress management, enough sleep, and frequent physical activity. Small lifestyle adjustments can have profound implications on hormonal well-being.

Seeking Professional Guidance
Recognizing the intricacy of hormonal balance, consulting healthcare professionals such as endocrinologists, gynecologists, and nutritionists is vital for tailored assistance. They can conduct assessments, offer solutions, and monitor progress.

Hormones as Health Allies
Rather than considering hormones as adversaries, recognizing their roles places them as friends in the pursuit of good health. Empowering individuals with knowledge develops a proactive and educated attitude to well-being.

Conclusion: Navigating the Symphony of Hormones
In finishing our in-depth tour into the realm of hormones, we've exposed the nuances of their orchestration in the big symphony of the body. From the throbbing rhythms of insulin to the crescendos of thyroid hormones, each plays a key role in defining our health and well-being.

As we move on, armed with knowledge and appreciation for this hormonal dance, remember that understanding your body's symphony is a continuous journey. Embrace the uniqueness of your hormonal composition, and allow this knowledge to guide you toward a peaceful and vigorous life. The path ahead entails tuning into the delicate melodies of your body, acknowledging the cues it provides, and dancing in sync with the ever-evolving symphony of hormones. Here's to the intricate beauty within the symphony of hormones that makes you uniquely you.

1. The Truth About Hormones and Weight

Welcome to the educational voyage into the delicate dance between hormones and weight. In this chapter, we'll dig into the intriguing world of hormones, those microscopic messengers that exert amazing control over our bodies. Get ready to understand the reality of how hormones might influence our weight and, more importantly, learn empowered techniques to attain harmony within.

The Hormonal Symphony
Imagine your body as a symphony, and hormones as the conductors ensuring that every instrument does its part. Insulin, cortisol, estrogen, and progesterone are the key players in this orchestra, each with a particular role in maintaining equilibrium.

Insulin: The Blood Sugar Maestro
Our journey begins with insulin, the maestro of blood sugar management. When we consume carbohydrates, insulin orchestrates the absorption of glucose into cells for energy. However, too much-processed sugar and refined carbs can lead to insulin resistance, upsetting the balance and promoting weight gain.
Tip: Opt for complex carbohydrates like whole grains and sweet potatoes to keep insulin levels in check.

Cortisol: The Stress Conductor
Cortisol, the stress hormone, takes center stage as life gets chaotic. While it's vital for survival, chronic stress can boost cortisol levels, urging the body to accumulate fat especially around the waist. Managing stress isn't just about peace of mind; it's a vital component in weight management.
Tip: Incorporate stress-reducing methods like deep breathing, meditation, or a leisurely walk into your daily routine.

Estrogen and Progesterone: The Hormonal Ballet
Ladies, this one's for you. Estrogen and progesterone, the dynamic couple, dance during your menstrual cycle, altering metabolism and water retention. Hormonal abnormalities, particularly during perimenopause, or disorders like polycystic ovarian syndrome (PCOS), might throw a curveball into your weight management attempts.
Tip: Chart your menstrual cycle and modify your food and workout program to its natural regularity.

Decoding the Weight-Hormone Connection
Understanding the hormonal subtleties is only part of the puzzle. Let's explore the facts about how these hormones can affect weight and what you can do about it.

Hormonal Havoc and Cravings
Ever wondered why stress makes you seek comfort foods? Cortisol, our stress conductor, can induce desires for sugary and greasy treats, leading to emotional eating. Recognizing this relationship helps you to pick healthier coping techniques.
Tip: Swap the candy for a brisk walk or a talk with a friend when stress arises.

Insulin and the Sugar Rollercoaster
Too much-refined carbohydrates can put insulin on a rollercoaster ride, leading to energy dumps and additional cravings. The idea is to maintain stable blood sugar levels by choosing complex carbohydrates and including protein and fiber in your meals.
Tip: Snack on nuts, seeds, or veggies with hummus for prolonged energy.

The Menstrual Weight Mystery
Ladies, your menstrual cycle may alter the scale, with water retention and metabolic variations having a part. Instead of stressing over these momentary shifts, accept the ebb and flow of your body's natural rhythm.
Tip: Stay hydrated and focus on fueling your body with complete, nutrient-dense foods during your period.

Nurturing Hormonal Harmony
Now that you're armed with the knowledge of the weight-hormone connection, it's time to go on a road toward hormonal equilibrium.

Mindful Eating
 Mindful eating helps you create a healthier connection with food, minimizing emotional eating driven by hormonal swings.
Tip: Take time before meals to appreciate the colors, textures, and flavors on your plate.

Hormone-Friendly Workouts
Tailor your exercise routine to assist hormonal balance. Incorporate a mix of aerobic, strength training, and activities like yoga to enhance general well-being.
Tip: Find activities you enjoy to make exercise a sustainable part of your routine.

Rest and Rejuvenate
Quality sleep is non-negotiable for hormonal equilibrium. Aim for 7-9 hours of unbroken sleep each night to maintain your body's natural cycle.
Tip: Create a bedtime ritual, reduce the lights, and power down electronic devices an hour before sleep.

Embrace Your Hormonal Wisdom

As we complete this chapter, remember that your body is a beautifully complicated system, finely adjusted by hormones. By understanding their influence on weight and adopting hormone-friendly practices, you may empower yourself to navigate this delicate dance with grace and confidence. Embrace your hormonal knowledge, and let it guide you on the path to lifelong well-being.

2. The Marvel of Leanness: Unveiling the Role of Growth in Weight Maintenance

Welcome to a chapter that unveils the secret dance between growth and leanness. In this research, we'll dive into the interesting interplay of biological processes that contribute to keeping a slim and healthy physique. Prepare to be astonished by the various dynamics at play and discover how nurturing development can be your ally on the route to lifelong leanness.

The Dynamic Symphony of Growth
Imagine your body as a thriving garden, and growth as the sunlight that fuels its vitality. Growth is not only about getting taller; it's a constant process that repairs, renews, and optimizes various systems within your body.

Building Blocks of Growth
At the heart of growth lies the complicated dance of proteins, amino acids, and hormones. When you engage in activities that drive development whether it's through exercise, a nutrient-rich diet, or adequate sleep you provide your body with the vital building blocks it needs to thrive.
Tip: Prioritize protein-rich foods like lean meats, beans, and nuts to feed your body's development machinery.

Leanness and Metabolic Marvels
Now, let's explore the connection between growth and the marvel of metabolic efficiency that contributes to preserving leanness.

Muscle, Metabolism, and Leanness
Muscle is not just about strength; it's a metabolic powerhouse. The more lean muscle mass you have, the more effectively your body burns calories at rest. Engaging in resistance training, such as weightlifting or bodyweight exercises, becomes a crucial actor in stimulating muscle growth and sustaining leanness.
Tip: Incorporate strength training workouts into your regimen 2-3 times a week to contour your physique and enhance your metabolism.

The Energetic Efficiency of Growth
When your body is in a state of growth, it becomes a proficient energy-burning machine. This doesn't mean you have to be in a permanent state of growth, but including periods of focused growth, and activities can help to an overall more efficient metabolism.
Tip: Consider periodic stages of muscle-building workouts to kickstart growth-oriented metabolic processes.

Nutritional Support for Growth and Leanness
The link between growth and leanness extends to the plate. What you eat plays a critical function in providing the fuel necessary for your body's growing activities.

Nutrient-Rich Choices
Choosing a diet rich in vitamins, minerals, and antioxidants aids cellular growth and repair. Include a diverse array of fruits and veggies to ensure you're getting a spectrum of nutrients that contribute to general well-being.
Tip: Aim for a diverse and colorful meal, combining a mix of fruits and vegetables.

Protein Power
Protein isn't only for bodybuilders it's a crucial component in the growth game. Adequate protein consumption helps muscle repair, rehabilitation, and the synthesis of new tissues.
Tip: Include protein-rich items such as fish, poultry, tofu, and lentils in your meals.

The Growth Mindset
Leanness isn't only a physical state; it's a mindset. Cultivating a growth mentality extends beyond the physiological world into the mental and emotional dimensions of your well-being.

Positive Habits for Growth
Embrace the principle of constant improvement. Establish positive habits that contribute to your growth path, whether it's learning a new skill, practicing mindfulness, or fostering connections with supportive communities.
Tip: Set tiny, achievable goals to foster a mindset of ongoing growth and improvement.

Celebration of Your Growth Journey
    As we complete this chapter, remember that your road to leanness is not just about dropping pounds; it's a celebration of progress in every element of your being. By recognizing the symbiotic relationship between development and leanness and embracing the practices that support both, you're building the path for a vibrant, thriving, and leaner. Cheers to the marvel of growth and the boundless possibilities it uncovers on your way to sustainable leanness!

3. Testosterone Unveiled: Breaking Stereotypes and Embracing Balance

Welcome to the interesting world of testosterone, the hormone that has typically been identified with men yet holds great importance for both genders. In this chapter, we'll dive into the different roles of testosterone, refute popular beliefs, and explore how maintaining a balance of this hormone is vital for overall well-being. Get ready to shatter misconceptions and admire the delicate dance of testosterone in the human body.

Beyond the Stereotype: Testosterone in Women
Contrary to popular assumption, testosterone is not an exclusive club for guys. Women generate and require this hormone also, although at smaller levels. Testosterone is necessary for both genders, influencing several physiological functions that contribute to vitality and health.

Testosterone in Men: More than Muscle
For men, testosterone is frequently connected with muscle development and athletic strength. While it undoubtedly plays a critical role in growing and maintaining muscular mass, its influence goes far beyond the gym.
Tip: Engage in regular strength training workouts to boost healthy testosterone levels and overall well-being.

Testosterone in Women: Vital for Balance
In women, testosterone contributes to libido, energy levels, and the maintenance of bone density. Achieving hormonal balance is critical for women of all ages, from supporting reproductive health to navigating the changes associated with menopause.
Tip: Prioritize a nutrient-rich diet, frequent exercise, and stress management for hormonal equilibrium.

The Symphony of Hormones: Testosterone's Partners
Testosterone doesn't operate in isolation; it's part of a symphony of hormones that combine to regulate numerous biological activities. Understanding this interwoven dance offers light on the precise balance required for optimal health.

Estrogen and Testosterone: Dance Partners in Harmony
In women, estrogen and testosterone maintain a delicate tango. While estrogen is frequently associated with femininity, a healthy interplay between estrogen and testosterone is crucial for reproductive health, mood management, and overall vitality.
Tip: Nourish your body with a varied range of foods to assist the harmonious dance of estrogen and testosterone.

Testosterone and Cortisol: Balancing Act
Stress, the arch-nemesis of hormonal equilibrium, can alter testosterone levels. Chronic stress boosts cortisol, which, in turn, can interfere with the creation of testosterone. Managing stress becomes a vital element of keeping a balanced hormonal profile.
Tip: Prioritize stress-reducing activities such as meditation, deep breathing, or spending time in nature.

Lifestyle Choices for Optimal Testosterone Health
Now that we've identified the various roles of testosterone in both men and women, let's study lifestyle choices that encourage optimal hormonal health.

Nutrition for Testosterone Support
Your diet has a crucial role in ensuring healthy testosterone levels. Incorporate foods rich in zinc, vitamin D, and omega-3 fatty acids to give the necessary building blocks for testosterone production.
Tip: Include sources including lean meats, nuts, seeds, fatty fish, and fortified dairy in your diet.

Exercise: A Testosterone Boost
Regular physical exercise, especially resistance training and high-intensity interval training (HIIT), might promote the production of testosterone.
Tip: Aim for at least 150 minutes of moderate-intensity activity or 75 minutes of vigorous-intensity exercise every week.

Embracing Testosterone Balance
    As we complete this chapter, let's embrace the idea that testosterone is not exclusive to men it's an essential part of the symphony of hormones that orchestrates health and energy for all. By maintaining a healthy lifestyle, making informed decisions, and defying stereotypes, you prepare the path for a harmonic dance of hormones within your body. Here's to honoring testosterone's many responsibilities and ensuring that its influence is a force for well-being in both men and women!

4. Navigating the Keto Dilemma: A Friendly Exploration of the Low-Carb Conundrum

In recent years, keto has grabbed the nutrition landscape by storm, promising weight loss, greater energy, and mental clarity. However, like every nutritional regimen, it comes with its own set of problems and dilemmas. Let's engage in a friendly exploration of the keto dilemma, unraveling its principles, potential benefits, and hazards.

The Keto Foundation: Understanding the Basics
Ketosis Unveiled
At the heart of the keto problem lies the concept of ketosis, a metabolic condition when the body primarily burns fat for fuel instead of carbohydrates. This change is induced by dramatically reducing carb intake and boosting fat ingestion. The result? The body creates ketones, which become the predominant energy source.
Tip: For optimal ketosis, aim to keep your daily carb intake below 50 grams, primarily drawing energy from healthy fats.

The Macronutrient Balance
Keto is recognized for its macronutrient distribution of high fat, moderate protein, and low carb. This particular ratio is designed to stimulate the body to enter and sustain ketosis.
Tip: Incorporate healthy fats like avocados, olive oil, nuts, and seeds into your meals while keeping a tight check on carb intake.

The Keto Dilemma Explored
Now, let's unravel the numerous components of the keto problem, putting light on both its potential benefits and considerations.

The Potential Benefits of Keto
Weight Loss Wonders
Many supporters commend keto for its potential to promote weight loss, especially in the first phases. The change to burning fat might lead to a quick drop in water weight and reduced hunger.
Tip: While weight loss may occur, it's vital to focus on long-term health rather than fast remedies.

Stable Energy Levels
Supporters of keto generally describe greater energy levels and enhanced mental clarity. The steady flow of energy from fats, particularly ketones, can contribute to more persistent and stable energy throughout the day.
Tip: Pay heed to your body's cues; energy levels may differ from person to person.

The Considerations of Keto

Nutrient Shortfalls

By strictly restricting specific dietary groups, especially fruits, whole grains, and legumes, keto might potentially lead to nutrient deficiencies. It's crucial to properly plan your meals to ensure you're addressing your body's micronutrient demands.

Tip: Consider seeing a nutritionist or dietitian to design a well-rounded keto food plan.

Sustainability Challenges

The rigorous nature of the keto diet can provide sustainability issues for some individuals. Social interactions, limited food options, and unexpected cravings may impair long-term adherence.

Tip: Find versions of keto that suit your preferences and lifestyle, making it more sustainable in the long run.

A Balanced Approach to Keto

As we negotiate the keto problem, it's vital to adopt a balanced approach that values health and well-being over rigorous dietary guidelines.

Mindful Food Choices

Embrace a conscious approach to dietary choices within the keto paradigm. Opt for nutrient-dense, whole meals to guarantee you're not just hitting your macronutrient targets but also giving your body with necessary vitamins and minerals.

Tip: Include a range of colorful veggies and lean protein sources to promote nutritional diversity.

Regular Health Check-Ins

Consider occasional health check-ins to monitor the influence of the keto diet on your general well-being. Monitor biomarkers, energy levels, and any potential adverse effects to make educated judgments regarding its fit for you.

Tip: Listen to your body and be open to adjustments based on how you feel.

Finding Your Nutritional Sweet Spot

In conclusion, the keto dilemma is a multifaceted path that demands serious consideration of individual preferences, health goals, and lifestyle. Whether you're drawn to the potential benefits of weight loss and enhanced energy or wrestling with the issues of nutrient deficiencies and sustainability, finding your nutritional sweet spot is crucial. Remember, there is no one-size-fits-all approach to nutrition, and the greatest nutritional decision is one that matches your particular needs and boosts your overall well-being. Here's to your health, happiness, and striking the right balance on your keto journey!

PART II: A Transformative Four-Week Guide to Hormonal Harmony

Welcome to a voyage of self-discovery and well-being as we embark on a four-week roadmap to achieving hormonal balance. In this chapter, we'll go deep into lifestyle alterations, nutritional techniques, and mindful practices aimed at building harmony within your hormonal orchestra. Get ready to uncover the transforming potential of understanding and optimizing your hormones for a more vibrant and balanced life.

Week 1: Hormone Awareness and Assessment

Day 1-3: Hormone Health Check-Up

Morning:Schedule an appointment with your healthcare physician for a full hormone assessment.

Afternoon: Begin a notebook documenting energy levels, mood, and any visible changes in your body.

Day 4-7: Understanding Your Hormones

Morning: Dive into studies on major hormones estrogen, progesterone, insulin, and cortisol.

Afternoon: Reflect on your lifestyle and identify any factors affecting your hormone balance.

Week 1 Goals: Create a Hormone Journal

Document daily feelings, energy levels, and important occurrences.

Initiate Stress Reduction Practices: Incorporate exercises like deep breathing or meditation.

Week 2: Building a Nutrient Foundation

Day 8-14: Hydration and Whole Foods

Morning: Increase regular water intake; aim for at least 8 glasses.

Afternoon: Focus on including full, nutrient-dense foods in your meals.

Day 15-21: Blood Sugar Regulation - Morning: Choose a protein-rich meal to regulate blood sugar.

Afternoon: Opt for complex carbs and fiber-rich foods to sustain energy.

Week 2 Goals:

Hydration Focus: Drink a glass of water before each meal.

Complete Foods Challenge: Experiment with a new complete food each day.

Week 3: Hormone-Friendly Nutrition

Day 22-28: Omega-3 Fatty Acids and Magnesium

Morning: Include omega-3-rich foods (fatty fish, flaxseeds) in your breakfast.

Afternoon: Integrate magnesium-rich foods (leafy greens, almonds) into your meals.

Day 29-30: Mindful Eating

Morning: Practice mindful eating; savor each meal without interruptions.

Afternoon: Reflect on how different cuisines make you feel.

Week 3 Goals:
Omega-3 Boost: Consume omega-3-rich foods three times this week.
Mindful Eating Challenge: Set aside 15 minutes for each meal without interruptions.

Week 4: Stress Management and Sleep Optimization
Day 31-35: Mindfulness Practices Morning: Start your day with 10 minutes of meditation.
Afternoon: Incorporate brief breaks for mindful breathing.
Day 36-40: Sleep Rituals
Morning: Create a soothing bedtime ritual.
Afternoon: Aim for 7-9 hours of sleep each night.
Week 4 Goals: Stress-Reducing Activities: Commit to at least one stress-reducing practice each day.
Sleep Hygiene: Implement a consistent sleep regimen, changing as needed.

Ongoing Maintenance:
Monthly Reflection: Evaluate Hormone Journal: Look for patterns or triggers.
Adjust as Needed: Fine-tune your regimen based on your body's responses.
Regular Health Check-Ins: Consult Healthcare Providers: Schedule periodic check-ups to assess hormonal balance.

General Tips:
Stay Hydrated: Water is a powerful ally for hormone balance.
Organic and Hormone-Free: Choose organic and hormone-free choices when possible.
Limit Processed Foods: Minimize intake of processed foods and refined sugars.

Congratulations on finishing this amazing four-week journey to hormonal equilibrium! By cultivating awareness, making thoughtful choices, and embracing beneficial behaviors, you've built the framework for prolonged well-being. Remember, your journey to hormonal balance is ongoing, and these practices are designed to be adaptable, responding to your particular needs and experiences. Here's to a life full of vitality, balance, and the joy of well-nurtured hormones!

5. Nourishing Your Body: A Comprehensive Guide on Foods You Should Consume for Optimal Well-Being

Welcome to a chapter dedicated to the skill of fueling your body with wholesome, nutrient-rich foods. In this comprehensive guide, we'll explore the broad assortment of foods that contribute to your general well-being. From brilliant fruits and vegetables to lean meats and heart-healthy fats, let's dive into the colorful world of food and explore how making informed choices can be a tasty and fulfilling adventure.

The Foundation of a Healthy Plate
Colorful Fruits and Vegetables
Morning: Start your day with a fruit salad or a bright smoothie.
Afternoon: Incorporate a variety of vegetables into your meal and dinner.
Tip: Aim for a rainbow of hues to ensure a wide range of vitamins, minerals, and antioxidants.

Whole Grains
Morning: Opt for full grain options like oats or whole wheat toast.
Afternoon: Choose quinoa, brown rice, or whole grain pasta as a base for your meals.
Tip: Whole grains give fiber and sustained energy, supporting digestive health.

Lean Proteins
Morning: Include sources like eggs, Greek yogurt, or plant-based proteins.
Afternoon: Incorporate lean meats, fish, tofu, or lentils into your lunches and dinners.
Tip: Protein is needed for muscle repair, immunological function, and general satiety.

Healthy Fats
Morning: Add avocado or nuts to your breakfast.
Afternoon: Cook with olive oil and nibble on nuts for healthy fats.
Tip: Healthy fats enhance brain health, hormone production, and food absorption.

Foods for Specific Health Goals
Heart-Healthy Choices Morning: Oats with berries for soluble fiber.
Afternoon: Fatty fish (salmon, mackerel) for omega-3 fatty acids.
Tip: Prioritize foods rich in omega-3s, fiber, and antioxidants for heart health.

Bone Health Boosters
Morning: Fortified cereals or dairy for vitamin D and calcium.
Afternoon: Leafy greens and almonds for magnesium.
Tip: Support bone health with a mix of vitamin D, calcium, and magnesium-rich foods.

Immune System Support
Morning:Citrus fruits for vitamin C. Afternoon: Garlic and ginger in meals for immune-boosting characteristics.
Tip: A balanced diet with a range of vitamins and minerals supports a robust immune system.

Mindful Eating Practices
Hydration Heroes
Morning: Start your day with a glass of water.
Throughout the Day: Sip on herbal teas and keep a water bottle available.
Tip: Staying hydrated is vital for digestion, energy, and overall well-being.

Portion Control
Morning: Use smaller plates to avoid overeating.
Afternoon: Listen to your body's hunger and fullness cues.
Tip: Mindful portion control encourages balanced eating and minimizes excessive caloric intake.

Making Informed Choices
Organic and Locally Sourced
Morning: Choose organic fruits and vegetables wherever possible.
Afternoon: Support local farmers and markets for fresh products.
Tip: Organic and locally sourced foods may have better nutrient content and fewer pesticides.

Limiting Processed Foods
Morning: Opt for homemade breakfast options.
Afternoon: Choose whole foods over processed snacks.
Tip: Minimizing processed foods decreases additional sugars, salt, and bad fats.

Customizing Your Nutritional Journey
Personalized Nutrition
Morning: Consider any unique dietary requirements or preferences.
Afternoon: Explore new dishes and integrate variety into your meals.
Tip: Tailor your nutritional choices to suit your particular health objectives and preferences.

Seeking Professional Guidance
Morning: Research and identify credible nutritionists or dietitians.
Afternoon:Schedule a consultation to build a personalized nutrition plan.
Tip: Professional counsel guarantees you obtain advice tailored to your unique needs.

Cultivating a Joyful Relationship with Food
Mindful Mealtime Rituals
Morning: Create a pleasant breakfast environment.

Afternoon: Enjoy your meals without distractions.
Tip: Savoring your meals enriches the whole experience and promotes attentive eating.

 Celebrating Food Diversity
Morning: Explore international cuisines for breakfast options.
Afternoon: Incorporate a range of cultural foods into your weekly meal.
Tip: Diverse meals offer a spectrum of nutrients and flavors in your diet.

Reflecting on Your Nutritional Journey
Daily Journaling
Morning: Take time to reflect on your eating choices.
Afternoon: Note any changes in energy levels, mood, or digestion.
Tip: Journaling helps you become more attentive to your food habits and their effects.

Periodic Assessments
Morning: Schedule monthly assessments of your nutritional decisions.
Afternoon: Adjust your diet based on your goals and well-being.
Tip: Periodic assessments ensure your nutritional choices correspond with your growing health needs.

Closing Thoughts: A Journey of Culinary Delight
As we conclude our in-depth investigation of foods you should consume, remember that nourishing your body is not a restricting undertaking but a pleasant adventure. Embrace the multitude of choices available and savor the flavors, textures, and nourishment each meal delivers. By making informed decisions, tailoring your nutritional approach, and creating a good relationship with food, you're not simply sustaining your body you're partaking in a fascinating gastronomic experience. Here's to a life filled with robust health, tasty meals, and the delight of nourishing your body from the inside out!

6. Embracing Circadian Fasting, Unveiling Detoxification, and Troubleshooting with a Friendly Touch

Welcome to a chapter that tackles the potent trinity of circadian fasting, cleansing, and troubleshooting a holistic approach to maximizing your well-being. In the pleasant spirit of this guide, we'll go into the nuances of matching your eating patterns with your body's natural rhythms, understanding detoxification processes, and addressing frequent issues with a positive perspective. Let's start on a journey of well-being that spans the lovely dance of circadian fasting, the science of detoxification, and practical troubleshooting suggestions.

The Harmony of Circadian Fasting
Understanding Circadian Rhythms - Morning: Learn about your body's internal clock and how it affects numerous physiological functions.
Afternoon: Identify your normal peak energy and alertness intervals.
Tip: Tailor your eating window to fit with your circadian rhythms for increased energy and digestion.

Circadian Fasting Protocols
Morning: Explore common fasting regimens like the 16/8 or 14/10.
Afternoon: Consider your lifestyle and choose a fasting window that suits your routine.
Tip: Gradually ease into circadian fasting to allow your body to adapt comfortably.

The Art of Detoxification
 Unveiling Detox Myths
Morning: Debunk common myths regarding detox diets.
Afternoon: Understand the liver's involvement in natural detoxifying processes.
Tip: Focus on supporting your body's natural detox mechanisms through lifestyle choices.

Detox-Friendly Foods
Morning: Include cruciferous veggies like broccoli and kale in your meals.
Afternoon: Hydrate with water, herbal teas, and antioxidant-rich beverages.
Tip: Choose complete, nutrient-dense foods that help your body's detox pathways.

 Troubleshooting Your Wellness Journey
Common Challenges
Morning: Acknowledge potential obstacles like cravings or energy fluctuations.
Afternoon: Develop techniques to manage problems without getting discouraged.
Tip: Approach problems as chances for growth and positive change.

Mindful Eating Practices
Morning: Practice gratitude before meals. Afternoon: Listen to your body's hunger and fullness cues.
Tip: Mindful eating creates a more intuitive and joyful relationship with food.

Troubleshooting Digestive Concerns
Gut Health
Morning: Integrate probiotic-rich foods like yogurt or fermented veggies.
Afternoon: Prioritize fiber from fruits, vegetables, and whole grains.
Tip: Gradually increase fiber consumption to support a healthy gut microbiome.

Hydration Habits
Morning: Drink a glass of water upon waking.
Afternoon: Stay hydrated with infused water or herbal teas throughout the day.
Tip: Hydration promotes digestion and supports general cleansing processes.

Troubleshooting Energy Levels
Balanced Nutrition
Morning: Ensure meals have a balance of macronutrients protein, fats, and carbohydrates.
Afternoon: Snack on energy-boosting items like almonds or fruits.
Tip: Consistent, balanced nutrition helps maintain consistent energy levels.

Adequate Sleep
Morning: Establish a calming nighttime ritual.
Afternoon: Prioritize 7-9 hours of quality sleep each night.
Tip: Quality sleep is vital to general well-being and energy levels.

Celebrating Progress and Mindset Shifts
Reflecting on Your Journey
Morning: Journal about positive changes you've noticed.
Afternoon: Celebrate your victories, no matter how minor.
Tip: Cultivate a mindset of thankfulness and self-compassion throughout your wellness journey.

Altering and Evolving
Morning: Stay open to altering your strategy based on your experiences.
Afternoon: Embrace the mobility of your wellness path.
Tip: Your requirements and tastes may evolve be flexible and adaptable.

Final Thoughts: A Holistic Symphony of Well-Being

As we close this in-depth investigation, remember that embracing circadian fasting, comprehending detoxification, and troubleshooting with a gentle touch is a comprehensive symphony of well-being. Your body is a magnificent creature, capable of resilience and adaptation. By aligning with its natural rhythms, fueling it with whole meals, and diagnosing difficulties with a positive mindset, you're not simply maximizing your health you're building a lifetime of enduring well-being. Here's to the beautiful dance of circadian fasting, the knowledge of detoxification, and the happy troubleshoots that lead to a vibrant and harmonious life!

7. Crafting Your Culinary Symphony: A Comprehensive Guide to Meal Plans and Delectable Recipes for Hormonal Harmony

Welcome to the heart of your transforming journey where the science of hormonal balance meets the art of culinary delight. In this comprehensive chapter, we'll go deep into the intricate nuances of developing meal plans that correspond with your hormonal blueprint. From stimulating breakfasts to cozy evenings, we'll explore a broad selection of foods that not only nourish your body but also provide joy to your taste senses. Get ready to turn your kitchen into a haven of hormone-friendly recipes that make the four-week journey both delicious and rewarding!

The Magic of Breakfasts
The Morning Ritual (Weeks 1-2)
Mornings set the tone for the day, and your breakfast should be a harmonic blend of protein, healthy fats, and carbohydrates. Consider a wonderful Greek yogurt parfait covered with fresh berries, chia seeds, and a sprinkle of granola. The mix of protein and fiber will deliver a constant release of energy, maintaining your hormonal balance.
Tip: Experiment with different fruits and seeds to add diversity and maximum nutritional benefits.

Evolution of Energy (Weeks 3-4)
As your journey progresses, enhance your mornings with a nutrient-packed green smoothie. Blend spinach, banana, almond milk, and a scoop of protein powder for a refreshing and invigorating start to your day. The greens contribute to a vitamin-rich powerhouse, aiding in hormonal support and general health.
Tip: Customize your smoothie with ingredients that resonate with your taste preferences.

Lunchtime Symphony
The Vibrant Salad (Weeks 1-2)
Lunchtime calls for a vivid salad that not only thrills your palette but also supplies a spectrum of nutrients. Create a kale and quinoa salad with grilled chicken, cherry tomatoes, avocado, and a splash of balsamic vinaigrette. This ensemble offers a perfect balance of proteins, healthy fats, and complex carbohydrates.
Tip: Prep your items in advance to streamline your lunchtime routine.

Exploring Bowls of Goodness (Weeks 3-4)
Transition into weeks 3-4 with innovative lunch bowls. Consider a Mediterranean-inspired bowl including falafel, hummus, quinoa, and a mix of vibrant veggies. This not only satiates your taste buds but also supplies a varied assortment of nutrients needed for hormonal balance.

Tip: Don't shy away from experimenting with various grains, proteins, and dressings.

Energizing Snack Breaks
Nutty Nourishment (Weeks 1-2)
When the afternoon lull arrives, turn to a handful of mixed nuts and a piece of fruit for a nutrient-dense and fulfilling snack. The mix of protein, healthy fats, and natural carbohydrates will assist in maintaining stable blood sugar levels and keep energy consistent.
Tip: Pre-portion snacks to avoid mindless overeating.

Berry Bliss (Weeks 3-4)
Weeks 3-4 introduce a snack that honors the sweetness of nature a small dish of mixed berries complemented by a dollop of Greek yogurt. This refreshing choice delivers antioxidants, fiber, and a touch of protein for a tasty and beneficial pick-me-up.
Tip: Explore local farmer's markets for fresh, seasonal berries.

Crafting Dinner Delights
Salmon Serenity (Weeks 1-2)
Dinner should be a blend of flavors and nutrients that unwind your day. Try a baked salmon fillet combined with quinoa and a serving of steamed broccoli. Salmon provides omega-3 fatty acids to the table, adding to hormonal health and overall well-being.
Tip: Experiment with different herbs and spices to increase the taste.

Stir-Fry Symphony (Weeks 3-4)
Embrace the weeks ahead with a vegetable and shrimp stir-fry served over cauliflower rice. This low-carb alternative brings a variety of textures and colors, delivering a nutrient-rich and delicious dining experience.
Tip: Play with a spectrum of vegetables to make your stir-fry visually appealing.

Evening Elixirs and Dessert Dreams
Tranquil Teatime (Throughout the Weeks)
Evenings call for a moment of serenity. Wind down with a cup of herbal tea, such as chamomile or lavender. These teas not only calm your senses but also contribute to relaxation, promoting a tranquil environment for better sleep.
Tip: Create a calming routine around your teatime to increase its soothing effects.

Berry Bonanza (Throughout the Weeks)
Satisfy your sweet taste with a small bowl of mixed berries as a pleasant and wholesome dessert alternative. Berries are rich in antioxidants and natural sweetness, making them a wonderful treat that coincides with your hormonal goals.
Tip: Consider pouring a touch of honey for extra sweetness.

Customizing Your Culinary Adventure
Personalization Principles
As you move through the weeks, feel inspired to personalize your meals. Adjust portion sizes, experiment with different cooking techniques, and add seasonal food to keep your meals engaging and aligned with your preferences.
Tip: Keep a culinary journal to document your favorite recipes and adaptations.

Inviting Variety
Invite variety into your meals by discovering other cuisines and flavors. Incorporate a mix of herbs, spices, and condiments to keep your taste receptors engaged. The world of culinary inquiry is enormous, and your kitchen is your canvas.
Tip: Challenge yourself to try one new item or recipe each week.

Troubleshooting Tastes and Adjusting
Flavor Mastery
Don't be afraid to experiment with flavors. Herbs like basil, rosemary, and thyme, together with spices such as cumin, coriander, and turmeric, can change your food. Adjusting salt, acidity, or sweetness according to your taste preferences allows you to master the art of flavor.
Tip: Create your spice blends for a personalized touch.

Time Management Triumphs
Efficiency in the kitchen is crucial, especially during hectic days. Plan your meals, batch-cook staples like grains and meats, and explore time-saving cooking techniques. A well-organized kitchen boosts your capacity to cook hormone-friendly feasts without worry.
Tip: Designate a specific day for meal prep to set yourself up for success.

Celebrating Your Culinary Triumphs
Weekly Reflections
At the end of each week, take time to reflect on the flavors, textures, and emotions related to your meals. Consider sharing your favorite recipes and culinary discoveries with friends, and family, or even in a food journal. Celebrate the thrill of fueling your body and delighting your taste buds.
Tip: Create a weekly ritual of trying a new recipe or revisiting a beloved one.

Embracing Culinary Creativity
Cultivate a mindset of culinary innovation and enjoy the joy of cooking. Your kitchen is a canvas, and each meal is an opportunity to express yourself. Whether it's a simple breakfast or an elaborate feast, imbue your dishes with love and intention.
Tip: Share your culinary adventure on social media for inspiration and connection.

Closing Thoughts: A Feast for Hormonal Harmony

As we wind up this extended investigation of meal plans and recipes, remember that every dish you cook is an opportunity to nourish your body, support hormonal balance, and revel in the joy of flavorful experiences. The four-week trip ahead isn't just about reducing weight it's about celebrating the remarkable synergy between your nutritional choices and your well-being. Here's to savoring every taste, relishing each culinary invention, and embracing the lively symphony of hormone-harmonizing feasts on your way to a healthier, happier you.

Conclusion: A Culmination of Hormonal Harmony and Well-Being

As we reach the finish of our complete trip through the blueprint for achieving hormonal balance and weight loss, it's time to reflect on the revolutionary route you've gone on. Over the last chapters, we've investigated the intricate interplay between diet, hormones, and well-being, developing a roadmap personalized to empower and elevate you. Now, let's reduce the core of this voyage into a few important reflections.

Embracing Hormonal Balance
In delving into the nuances of hormonal balance, we've revealed the necessity of recognizing your body's cycles, honoring its signals, and embracing lifestyle choices that create peace. From the gentle practice of circadian fasting to the nourishing power of various, hormone-friendly foods, you've prepared yourself with information to assist your body's intrinsic ability to establish equilibrium.

Nourishing the Body, Mind, and Soul
The trip through meal plans and scrumptious recipes was more than a culinary exploration it was a celebration of sustenance at its finest. By crafting meals that correspond with your hormonal blueprint, you've not only embraced the science of nutrition but also elevated your relationship with food to a realm of joy, creativity, and self-care.

A Mindful Approach to Well-Being
Beyond the subtleties of diet and hormones, we've emphasized the role of mindfulness in your well-being journey. From growing awareness of your body's signals to fixing issues with a positive outlook, you've constructed a tapestry of mindfulness that goes beyond the plate to the greater canvas of your life.

Your Ongoing Journey
As you carry this blueprint forward into your daily life, remember that this is not a hard set of rules but a flexible guide designed to adapt to you. Your road toward hormonal balance and weight loss is uniquely yours, and the blueprint acts as a companion a supporting foundation upon which you can construct a sustainable, thriving lifestyle.

Celebrating Progress and Embracing Joy
Take a minute to celebrate your achievements, both great and small. Whether it's the newfound energy in your step, the tasty dishes that have become staples in your kitchen, or the mindfulness practices that have anchored you, each step forward is a win worth appreciating.

Your Health, Your Joy

Ultimately, the blueprint for hormonal balance and weight loss is a tool for your well-being, a roadmap to help you towards a better and happier you. As you continue on your journey, may you find joy in every good meal, strength in each thoughtful choice, and fulfillment in the continual discovery of what helps your body thrive.

Here's to the glowing health, the harmony of hormones, and the wonderful dance of well-being that awaits you on this path. May your road be filled with nutritious moments, joyful discoveries, and an abundance of vitality. Cheers to you and the glorious chapters of well-being that lay ahead!

Acknowledgments

Embarking on the road of creating "Blueprint For Women, Diet, and Hormones: A Comprehensive Four-Week Guide to Achieve Hormonal Balance and Lose Weight" has been a joyful and collaborative undertaking. As I extend my thanks, I am reminded that this project would not have been possible without the support, inspiration, and efforts of many wonderful individuals.

Appreciation for the Collaborators:
To the Expert Contributors
A heartfelt thank you to the healthcare professionals, dietitians, and specialists who willingly contributed their knowledge and views, providing important expertise to the blueprint.

To the Readers and Testers
A particular appreciation to the dedicated readers and testers who embraced the blueprint, providing valuable comments and helping polish the text for optimum impact.

Gratitude for Supportive Networks
To Friends and Family: Thank you for your consistent encouragement, understanding, and patience during the numerous hours committed to study and writing.

To Colleagues and Mentors:
A heartfelt appreciation for the support, guidance, and collaborative attitude that have powered the creative process. Your guidance has been important in building this comprehensive handbook.

Recognition for the Community
To the Online Community, I offer my gratitude to the different online groups that promoted thoughtful debates, shared experiences and created a vibrant space for learning and growth.

Heartfelt Thanks to You
Your interest, devotion, and commitment to your well-being are the driving force behind this guide. It is my earnest desire that the blueprint serves as a beneficial companion on your journey to hormonal balance and weight loss.

In the spirit of gratitude, I extend my thanks to each person who played a role in bringing this handbook to existence. May the lessons presented within these pages help to your health, happiness, and a harmonious life.

With heartfelt thanks,

Elizabeth Kettner, MD

About the Author

Dr. Elizabeth Kettner is a passionate and motivated medical practitioner with a mission to inspire individuals on their journey to optimal health and well-being. With a wealth of expertise and experience in the field of medicine, Dr. Kettner has become a trusted authority on women's health, hormonal balance, and weight management.

Academic Excellence and Medical Expertise

Dr. Kettner got her Doctor of Medicine (MD) degree from a top medical institution in the USA, where her devotion to academic excellence and compassionate patient care set her apart. Throughout her medical school, she developed a particular interest in the complicated interplay between hormones, nutrition, and overall health.

Specialization in Women's Health

Driven by a desire to make a meaningful influence on the lives of women, Dr. Kettner chose to specialize in women's health. Her devotion to understanding the particular hormonal issues experienced by women at different life phases drove her to pursue advanced training and research in the field.

A Compassionate Healer and Advocate

Known for her empathic approach and tireless commitment to patient well-being, Dr. Kettner has played a crucial role in aiding individuals on their health journeys. She believes in a holistic approach to medicine, treating not just the physical aspects of health but also the emotional and psychological elements that contribute to total well-being.

Pioneering Hormonal Balance Research

Dr. Kettner's passion for expanding the understanding of hormonal balance has pushed her to actively engage in research. Her contributions to the field include important studies on the impact of lifestyle, nutrition, and circadian rhythms on hormonal health. Through her work, she seeks to bridge the gap between medical research and practical, actionable insights for those seeking hormonal equilibrium.

Authorship and Knowledge Sharing

Driven by a love for teaching and knowledge transmission, Dr. Kettner has produced numerous articles, and research papers, and contributed to medical publications. "Blueprint For Women, Diet and Hormones: A Comprehensive Four-Week Guide to Achieve Hormonal Balance and Lose Weight" stands as a tribute to her commitment to offering accessible and evidence-based information for anyone seeking dramatic health changes.

Engaging with the Community

Dr. Kettner regularly participates with her community through educational seminars, internet platforms, and speaking engagements. She acknowledges the importance of community support in creating health-conscious lifestyles and works to build spaces where individuals may share stories and learn from each other.

A Vision for Well-Being

Beyond her clinical practice, Dr. Elizabeth Kettner envisions a world where individuals are empowered to take care of their health, armed with knowledge, inspiration, and a feeling of community. Through her work, she continues to inspire and guide people on their paths to hormonal balance, weight management, and healthy well-being.

www.ingramcontent.com/pod-product-compliance
Lightning Source LLC
Chambersburg PA
CBHW060902260726

48661CB00008B/3410